Yoga for Chickens

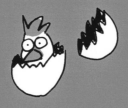

For Keith and Kai—my little chickadees

Yoga for Chickens

RELAXING YOUR INNER CHICK

or

Enlightened Poses Straight from the Coop

by Lynn Brunelle

CHRONICLE BOOKS

SAN FRANCISCO

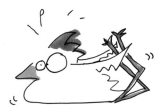

Special thanks to Meg Parsont and Lisa Campbell, who became one with the poses in this book. Without them, many of the translations would not have been possible. And thanks to Christine Carswell for her focus, humor, and enlightened spirit.

Library of Congress Cataloging-in-Publication Data is available.

ISBN: 0–8118–4311–4

Manufactured in China

Designed by Headcase Design • www.headcasedesign.com

Distributed in Canada by Raincoast Books
9050 Shaughnessy Street • Vancouver, British Columbia V6P 6E5

10 9 8 7 6 5 4 3 2 1

Chronicle Books LLC
85 Second Street • San Francisco, California 94105
www.chroniclebooks.com

TABLE OF CONTENTS

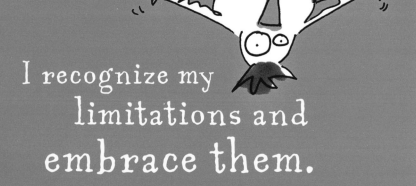

I recognize my limitations and embrace them.

A Word from the Coop

Feeling fried? All cooped up? Stressed out by the pecking order? If you feel like you've been laying a lot of eggs lately, Yoga for Chickens is the book for you.

Movie stars, business executives, health professionals—everybody's talking about what chickens have known for millions of years. Yoga encourages the mind, body, and spirit to become as one. It will help you transcend yourself. The exercises on these pages come from a long tradition of discovery and mindfulness, as practiced by the great yolkic masters and common fowl in barnyards and coops across time and continents.

Let me take you under my wing and share my bird-brained wisdom with you. Let me lead you along the poultry path of self-awareness and well-being. Learn to be present in the feathery flow of time from one moment to the next. Lay your worries aside and let your inner spring chicken begin to cluck. Let me soothe those ruffled feathers and guide you from your scrambled state to the organic sublimeness of Yoga for Chickens.

It's never too late to be a tender chicken in a tough world.

On Being and Chickenness

To be a chicken is a study—a meditation, if you will. There is such wisdom in the chicken yard! Perhaps you've seen us chickens, staring as if blankly into space. We are pondering the imponderables. The meaning of existence. We are being mindful.

Consider these simple joys of chickendom:

When the Sun Rises, Wake with a Song

Share the pure joy of rediscovering the world as you left it and declare the life-affirming elation of the returning sun, radiant like a yolk in the sky. Take nothing for granted. As chickens, we simply can't help but rejoice and crow into the morning air. Perhaps you've been annoyed in the past by the rooster's sun salutation. Crack open your assumptions and think again with new perspective (see page 94).

Search

From the moment the sun comes up, we are in constant search of enlightenment. Picking, scratching, digging, and pecking are all studied exercises of this longstanding tradition of exploration as well as the search for nourishment. By becoming more mindful of the source of our nourishment and enjoying the pathway of gathering, we grow the spirit.

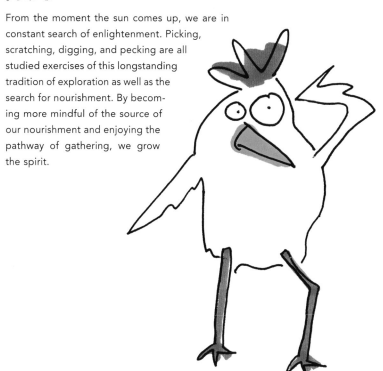

I accept all the universe offers me.

Embrace Dust

A roll in the dirt and a shake of the feathers is, on the surface, a fabulous cosmetic regimen. The minerals and complex compounds found in the most seemingly humble matter can, when applied daily, brighten the sheen of any hen's feathers. They bring luster and beauty to the flock and keep it bug free. But contemplate the deeper implications of this surface beauty. Embrace the very dust from which we all sprang! To immerse one's self in the mud of origin connects us spiritually to the planet, the creatures that live here, and our true selves.

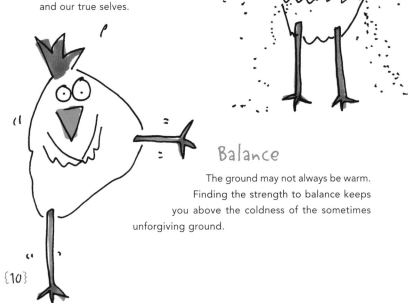

Balance

The ground may not always be warm. Finding the strength to balance keeps you above the coldness of the sometimes unforgiving ground.

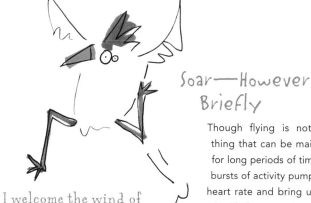

Soar—However Briefly

Though flying is not something that can be maintained for long periods of time, short bursts of activity pump up the heart rate and bring us closer to the life force we share with all living things. Leaving the ground for a few moments not only elevates the spirit, but also forces us to become more grounded. Each thud of an awkward landing is a conscious way of reconnecting with the solid, true energy of the earth.

I welcome the wind of life ruffling through my feathers.

Practice Stillness

Perch here and there. Luxuriate in a mindful, conscious presence. Grasp the physicality of the perch with every feather of your being as you dive deeper into your consciousness and release the unnecessary.

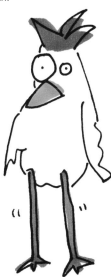

Release the Life Force

Lay an egg—two, if you're lucky—every day. Feel the release! Letting go is an essential element of finding joy.

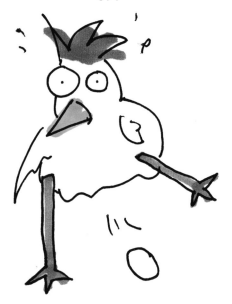

Draw from the Circle of Life

Acknowledge the inevitability of negative energy and pain. Be alert to foxes and snakes in the grass, but do not try to judge or change them. Find life-embracing meaning, even when the sky is falling.

Hatch a Plan

To get you off to a flying start, this book explores the yoga basics in four easy-to-follow sections:

Breathing
It's important.

Stretching
Turn up the heat with these must-do warm-ups.

Poses and postures
Learn the hard-boiled secrets of unruffling your feathers with poses in every position. You'll even find some to do with your partner that will really bring you out of your shell.

Chicken fix-it routines
Target problem areas of stress: wings, legs, thighs, etc.

As you practice your poses, listen to your body—pay attention to and be aware of your body. New sensations, sounds, and changes may surprise you. Don't worry. It's all part of the letting-go process.

Chickens' feathery down provides a nice comfy cushion for poses and stretches. Should you lack your own natural padding, feel free to use a mat.

Throughout this book, you'll find affirmations and profound meditations that have been passed down to us by the sages. Affirm your being and oneness! Ponder the riddles of the ages.

Which came first? The chicken or the egg?

A Joyful Noise—Cluck!

Chanting is an excellent way to burn tension and free the mind and spirit. There are days when the barnyard is abuzz with individual chantings: porcine oinks, equine whinnies, feline meows, canine woofs, and various aviary chirpings. It is truly the sound of all sounds and it sweeps away negative energy while cleansing and making way for total serenity. You have your own joyful noise. For chickens, the cluck is perfection.

There are four parts to the cluck:

- Ah
- Oh
- Mmm
- CLUCK!!!

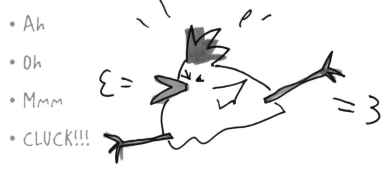

Make yourself comfortable. You can be sitting or standing. Close your eyes and breathe slowly and deeply. Concentrate on your inner chick and begin chanting. If you feel self-conscious, cluck silently to yourself until you feel the volume build. When you are ready, take a deep breath and let loose with the wild cluck from within. Repeat at least 10 times, or more often during egg laying.

The Object of Contemplation

The chicken is the symbol of perfection and simplicity. To meditate upon the chicken is to focus on the deep philosophical aspects of what yoga really means for the true seeker.

Look at this chicken either on the page or in your mind's eye when you practice and repeat the mantra, "Chickens are perfection." When your mind flies off, ground it again by invoking this image.

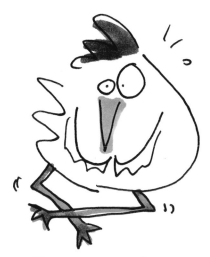

Chickens are perfection.

Breathe

It all begins with breathing. You take over 20,000 breaths a day. Why not make them work for you as deeply as possible? Proper breathing is the key to a satisfying yoga experience. It brings a new dynamism, a surge of energy to tired limbs. So rejoice in your chicken breath and thank the muscles in your diaphragm and lungs for moving so beautifully in synch with the universe.

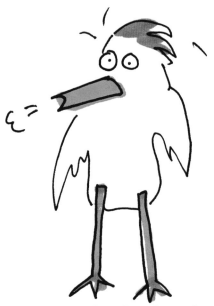

I breathe, therefore I live.

Observing the Breath

If you don't breathe, it's just not healthy. Take the time to really feel the breath move in and out of your body. This technique is great if you need a little personal space and the coop is a-clucking with activity. Move within and there's always "me time."

Sit cross-legged on the ground. Lay one wing on your belly and one on your heart. Feel deeply through the fluff and feather and concentrate on each breath. Close your eyes and move within. Breathe. Notice that you're breathing. Feel your feathers rise and fall. Be conscious of the moment and return to your breathing in preparation for the extended breathing exercises in the following pages.

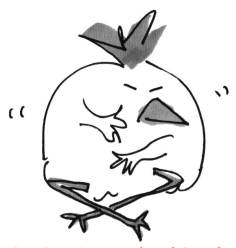

I am brand-new with each breath.

Wings like Bellows Breath

This breathing technique has been passed down to us by the great Asian masters, who have a long tradition of enjoying red-hot spicy peppers in their diet. It is unusual in yogic practice in that it calls for vigorous movement, which, combined with the wide-open eyes and almost frantic nature of the inhale and exhale, dispels any negative energy and brings any heat back down to a calm, collected self.

Stand with feet comfortably set apart. Open your eyes and your beak as wide as possible. Inhale deeply and fling out your open wings. Flap. Exhale and tuck your beak under, curl your tail feathers in, and bring the wings together at your wishbone. Repeat until you feel quite cool.

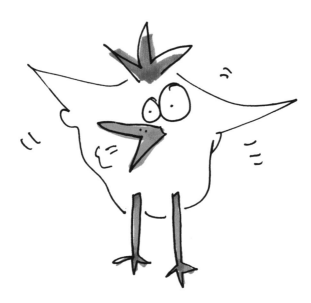

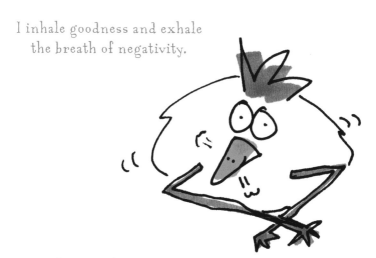

I inhale goodness and exhale the breath of negativity.

Laughing Chicken Breath

Another wisdom we have received from the ancients is that humor is life. After food, water, exercise, shelter, a healthy family, company, a good coop, protection from foxes and weasels, a caring farmer, and fresh straw, humor is essential. This breathing technique brings humor into the spiritual realm and allows the eternal laughter to cleanse and purify your being. A word of caution: You can laugh yourself dizzy with this exercise.

Sit comfortably on the ground. Take a deep breath in and hold it for a few seconds. As you exhale, contract your abdomen sharply so that it expels your breath in forceful little "ha!"s through your beak until all the breath has left your body. Repeat.

ANCIENT
CHICKEN KOANS
ko'an (kō'än) n. (Jap.) a paradoxical question

The word koan literally means "a public document." This actually has roots in chickenness. Our public display of practicing mindfulness has been on view on farms, coops, and yards for millions of years but only recently has any attention been drawn to our depth. Now, a koan has come to mean a form of pondering based on the actions of famous poultric masters. It is a baffling riddle with no answer, no logic, and no connection.

Ponder these imponderables:

Why did the chicken cross the road?

What is the sound of one wing flapping?

Which came first—the chicken or the egg?

Is an empty nest really empty?

Stretch

Before you start anything physical, you need to ready your body. The neck, thighs, and wings, in particular, should be gently stretched in preparation for your choice of pose. Chickens are constantly stretching, which is often mistaken for simple barn-yard activity. Never judge by appearances! The bobbing of the head, the rooster's extended strut, the unruffling of the feathers are just a few of our everyday warm-ups.

Gizzard Stretch

This stretch elongates your neck, increasing mobility and expressiveness. It also allows you to see things from a new perspective.

Stand straight with your wings down by your sides. Inhale and bring your head down to your right shoulder. Hold for a few seconds. Exhale and bring your head back up to the starting position. Bob briefly, being careful not to overextend the neck, to shake out the kinks. Repeat on your left side.

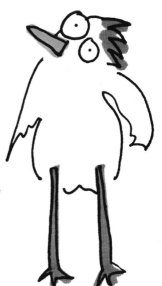

I Dunno Shoulder Shrug

A wonderful warm-up that, when done correctly, may be practiced beneficially throughout the day.

Stand straight with your wings down by your sides. Keep your beak facing straight ahead. Inhale and bring your shoulders up as far as possible, preferably in line with your beak if you can. Try not to strain—a blank look on your face increases the depth of this pose.

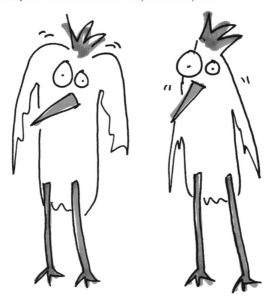

Exhale and release.

Hippie Chick

Perfect for working out kinks in your back, neck, and legs, this is a very grounding stretch that brings you close to the great Earth Mother. It also offers the perfect opportunity to feel the powerful force that gravity has on the body.

Sit on the ground with your legs straight out in front of you. Stretch your wings and reach for your toes. Pull your body forward and really stretch your wingtips and beak toward your feet, as if there's some grain just out of reach.

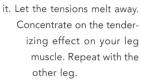

Drumstick Stretch

Tight thighs can leave you feeling burnt. A little stretch does wonders for clearing the juices.

Lie on the ground, legs straight out. Bring one knee into your breast and hug it. Let the tensions melt away. Concentrate on the tenderizing effect on your leg muscle. Repeat with the other leg.

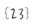

Cat-Cow

There is so much to be learned from those around us!
Each day in the farmyard brings fresh insights.
This combined stretch, which is particularly
good for the spine, was inspired by the
yoga practices of my fellow creatures.

Get down on all fours as if you were
a cat. Exhale and pull your back
up, up to the sky. Drop your
beak and tuck your tail under.
Embrace your fear of the pred-
ator! Meow! You're a cat!

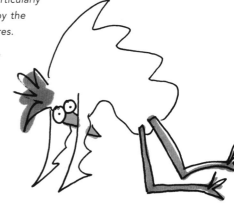

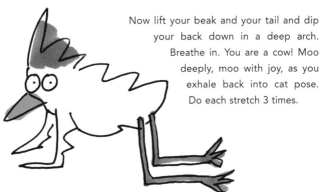

Now lift your beak and your tail and dip
your back down in a deep arch.
Breathe in. You are a cow! Moo
deeply, moo with joy, as you
exhale back into cat pose.
Do each stretch 3 times.

Flying Bug/Crawling Bug

Treats can come your way by many different means. Bugs, for example, can tantalize you by flying past or crawling by. This pose celebrates the joy of discovery—mid-air or mid-mud.

Stand straight, legs slightly apart, wings relaxed by your sides. Inhale and clasp your wings behind you. Point your beak up, arch your back, and thrust your breastbone to the sky. Look for flying bugs.

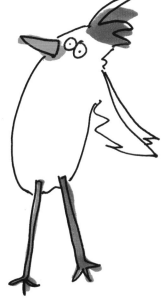

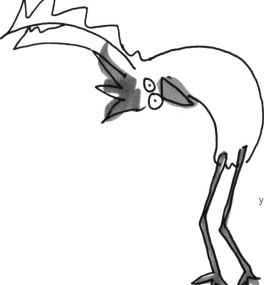

Exhale and tuck your breastbone under as you bring your beak and your focus to the ground. Keeping your wings together, allow them to fall over your comb as far as you can. Feel the stretch as you search for crawlers.

Standing Chicken Poses

This section begins with two poses that are key to many of the positions you'll be enjoying as you expand your yoga practice. A word to the wise about standing poses: Balancing can be tricky. Don't worry if you topple over. Feel no shame or humiliation. Simply pick yourself up, dust yourself off, and rejoice in starting all over again.

Weathervane

It all begins with this proud pose. Feel the energy flow from the ground through your strong legs into each and every sinew and out of every feather. Feel the wind whistle through your comb. You are alive! Start your yoga practice with this journey to mindfulness and continue to enjoy it between each of the standing poses.

Stand straight and tall, toes pointing forward, wings relaxed by your sides. Tuck in your tail feathers, raise your head up straight, beak forward, comb erect. Take a deep breath. Center yourself, release yourself to other forces. Imagine the wind is able to point you in any direction. You are at one with the powerful winds.

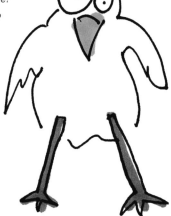

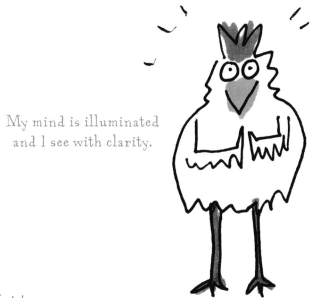

My mind is illuminated
and I see with clarity.

Wishbone

Another version of the Weathervane is the Wishbone. Joining the wings together at the wishbone chakra can add a little zip to the energy you're drawing from the ground.

Stand straight and tall, legs slightly apart, toes facing forward. Bring your wings up, then lower and join them prayerlike in front of your breastbone. This is a very sincere pose.

Over the Coop

We all dream. The barn, the coop, the fence—they can seem insurmountable, yet with concentration and practice, this elegant pose can help you transcend them in your mind.

Start in Weathervane pose (see page 26). Inhale and stretch your wings straight out at your sides. Look straight ahead and think lofty thoughts. Imagine flying above the coop. Hold for a count of 3 and exhale your wings down.

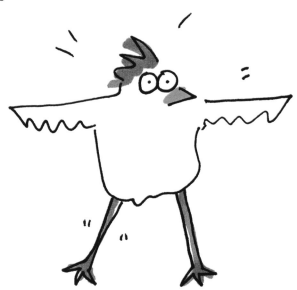

The universe applauds my journey.

Poultry Pose

Barbara Walters said it best when she asked, "If you were a tree, what kind of tree would you be?" The answer is obvious, isn't it? This pose stimulates balance and strength as well as the intellect.

Start in Weathervane pose (see page 26). Bend your left knee and tuck the sole of your foot under until it touches your right thigh (try not to let your toes gouge your leg). Stretch your wings out to the side and breathe in. You are a mighty oak!

Hold for a moment or two. Exhale. If you can keep your balance, inhale and stretch your wings to the sky. You are an ancient redwood!

Hold for a count of 3 and bring your wings down slowly, back into Wishbone pose (see page 27). Place your right foot back on the ground. Feel the energy of the earth surge through your roots. Repeat with the other leg.

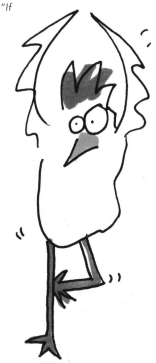

If I plant a feather, what will it grow?

Eagle

We must look to our fine feathered friends—and enemies—to learn more about ourselves and take another step in our path to fulfillment. This pose is inspired by a treacherous enemy that flies overhead and swoops to the coop to snack on unsuspecting chickens. Though she is feared, the eagle is strong and fierce. These are good qualities to enmesh into our own being. This pose is the physical manifestation of the twist in thinking one must embrace in order to become one with the enemy.

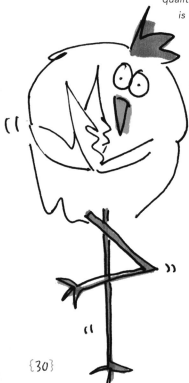

Stand with your feet a little apart. Inhale and raise your wings to shoulder height. Raise your right leg and wrap it behind and around the standing left leg. While you balance on one foot, wrap your left wing around your right in front of you. Breathe and stand there in this twisted position. Meditate upon how the bad can be good, how pain can become joy. Keep breathing. Release and repeat on the other side.

I embrace the power of
my beautiful body.

My body is a
conduit for joy.

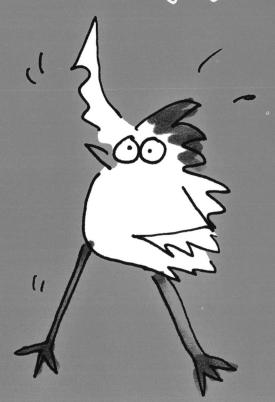

Chicken Feed Poses

Everyday routine can inspire yoga practice and bring unexpected joy. Morning comes and, as chickens, we begin our timeless search for grain, bugs, or tiny worms. A lazy chicken simply stands and pecks. But the mindful chicken takes the opportunity to strengthen the wing muscles and enhance the breast while also stretching and aligning the spine. Do these poses in sequence.

Grain on Ground Pose

Note how this position increases the ground viewing area to the rear.

From an all-fours position, tuck your toes under and straighten your legs. Exhale and point your tail feathers to the sky while reaching back with your heels, beak facing down and wings pressed to the ground. Feel the length along your spine. Feel the stretch in your thighs and tendons. Breathe in and out and meditate on all the wondrous things you can find on the ground in this position.

In the grain is infinity.

Moving Target Lunge

This pose is great for getting a head start on a moving meal.

Stand with your feet one wing's distance apart. Take a step back with your left leg and lift your head and breast. Feel the stretch, straighten it, bending your right knee in a lunge. Breathe.

I sink my beak into the
goodness of life.

Worm!

This is a whole-body strengthener that allows you to locate and devour the tastiest of nearby worms.

From the Moving Target Lunge (see above), lower your wingtips to the ground. Inhale. Step back with your right leg, straighten your body, and balance on your toes and the flats of your wingtips. Keep your body straight and your belly tight, and look out at the barnyard ahead of you. Hold for 3 seconds.

Exhale and hold this push-up position. Take a moment to view the bugs.

SHORT BEAK

Chicken held up her short beak and said, "If you call this a short beak, you oppose its reality. If you do not call it a short beak, you ignore the fact. Now what do you wish to call this?"

OLD PAIL

Chicken was unable to attain the fruits of meditation for a long time. At last one moonlit night in the barnyard, she was carrying water in an old pail. The bottom fell out of the pail, and at that moment Chicken was set free!

Peek Around the Fencepost

The inspiration for this all-body stretch came one morning when I was stuck in the mud of the farmyard—an incredibly grounding experience—and was mindful of the day's first feeding. The stability of my feet allowed me to stretch for a good view around the fencepost before me and wave my wings, signaling to the farmer that I was ready to accept his grain.

Start from the Wishbone pose (see page 27) and then stretch your wings overhead. Exhale and lean to the right. Inhale and return to center. Then exhale and lean to the left.

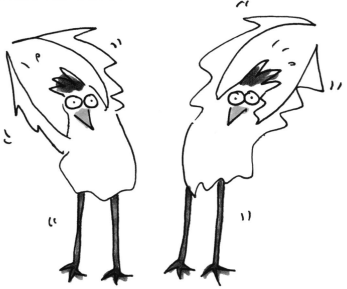

I honor the barnyard. It honors me.

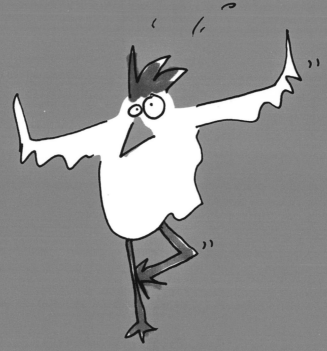

My stillness
moves through me
from the inside out.

One Wing Flapping

The following three poses are often done in sequence. This is not just because of their physical similarity, but also because they invite us to ponder deeply as we reach for the stars.

Stand with your feet one wing's distance apart. They should be wide, but stable. Turn your right leg at a right angle to your body and your left turned slightly pigeon-toed inward. Inhale and stretch your wings out to the sides. Bend over and place your right wingtip as far down as you can on your right leg. Raise your left wing up to the sky. As the breeze gently wafts your feathers, hold for several breaths and consider the sound of your left wing flapping. Reverse the pose.

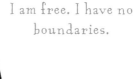

I am free. I have no boundaries.

Toe/Sky Pose

The stretch of your body in opposite directions can deliver the most sublime and powerful experience. This Toe/Sky Pose is a perfect example of the opposing stretch and the emotional and spiritual dichotomy of being grounded in the physical and seeking the metaphysical.

Stand with your feet one wing's distance apart. They should be wide, but stable. Turn your right leg at a right angle to your body and your left turned pointing straight ahead. Inhale and stretch your wings out to the sides. Bend your left knee. Reach up to the sky with your right wing while stretching down for your left toe with your left wing so that your wings form a straight diagonal. Feel the dichotomy of the two kingdoms of chicken—earth and sky. Breathe into it. Exhale and straighten up. Reverse the pose.

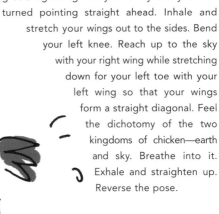

I am open to the soaring
and sinking of life.

It's a Bird! It's a Plane!

There is wisdom in confusion. Many times I have asked a question only to find deeper wisdom in the quest for an answer than in the answer itself. It may be a bird, it may be a plane, but this pose is about the physical process of asking.

Stand with your feet one wing's distance apart, wide, but stable. Turn your left leg at a right angle to your body and your right turned slightly pigeon-toed inward. Exhale and twist your body to the left, reaching up with both wings up to the sky. Try to keep your wing tips together. Bend your left leg and straighten your right to create a diagonal from tip to toe. Take several deep breaths as you focus your gaze and energy to the sky in an inquisitive manner. Imagine you feel your hard-working feet leave the ground. Exhale and return to center. Reverse the pose.

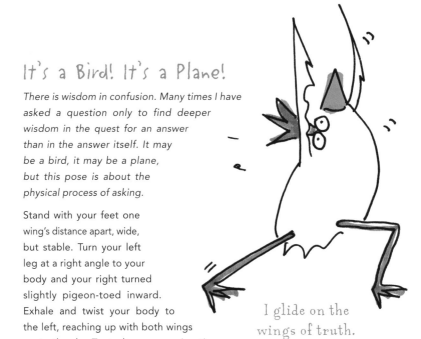

I glide on the wings of truth.

Chicken Surprise

Surprises can come in many different forms.

Begin in Weathervane pose (see page 26). Inhale and stretch your wings out in front of you, parallel to the ground. Exhale and bend your knees, slowly lowering your tail feathers, as if onto an imaginary nest. Hold your breath for a count of 3. Inhale back up to standing. This pose can help strengthen the body for egg laying as well as eliminate unwanted toxins.

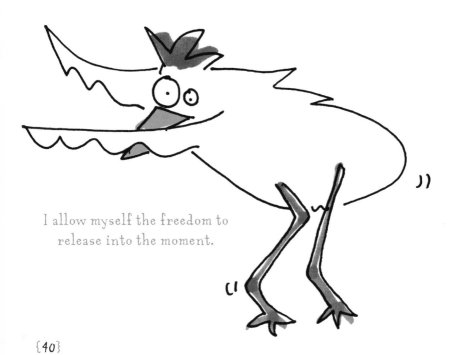

I allow myself the freedom to release into the moment.

MUDDY ROAD

Bantam and Chickido were once traveling together down a muddy road. A heavy rain was still falling. Coming around a bend, they met a lovely hen in silky feathers, unable to cross the intersection.

"Come on, little hen," said Bantam at once. Lifting her in his wings, he carried her over the mud.

Chickido did not cluck again until that night when they reached a friendly coop. Then he no longer could restrain himself. "We roosters don't go near hens," he told Bantam, "especially not young and lovely ones covered with silky feathers. It is dangerous. Why did you do that?"

"I left the hen there," said Bantam. "Are you still carrying her?"

Sitting Chicken Poses

There is no position that speaks more profoundly to the chicken than to sit. At the most subliminal level, it takes us back to the nest from which we all sprang, brought to hatching by our mothers' warmth and patient brooding. All of these poses are informed by the depths of such subconscious memories.

Egg Laying Pose

This nurturing pose taps into the great power that is motherhood. Great power and pain. In this pose you are connecting your creation energy with the life force of the earth, with all that implies.

Find a comfortable place to sit and place your tailfeathers directly on the ground. Fold your legs in front of you so that your left leg is resting on the ground and your right leg is resting on your left thigh (if you can get there!), feet as close to your body as possible. Sit up straight and place your wingtips together. Feel the life-giving energy flow from the ground through your tailfeathers and course throughout your body. Feel it nurture your private self.

Parson's Nose to the Grindstone

Sometimes after a hard day you just feel all tied up in knots, don't you? This is a super pose for disentangling the stress.

Start in Egg Laying Pose (see facing page). Wrap your right wing around your left knee and cradle it to your breast. Take yourself under your wing; absorb the nurturing energy from your own breast. Exhale and twist your body to the left, placing your left wingtips on the ground. Exhale and release. Repeat on your other side.

Ground Chicken

Even though our bodies are very much influenced by gravity, our minds can ring through the air like a clap of thunder! Rest your body with this pose between more vigorous postures.

From a kneeling position, inhale and reach up with both wings. Keep your tailfeathers grounded and reach your comb skyward. Your beak should face forward. Feel your spine lengthen and your spirit lighten.

I yield to the earth.

Crow

Since the crow is such a trickster, this pose is an editorial comment on what we think of his pranks. The pose is a pensive one that requires great strength and fortitude.

Starting on all fours, bend your legs and place them outside your wings. Slowly lift your legs up into the air, so that your lower leg is resting on your upper wings and your legs are roughly parallel to the ground. Gaze forward and feel your balance transfer from your feet to your wings. Wave your tailfeathers to the sky in a salute to crow humor. Exhale and release back to the ground. Repeat as strength allows.

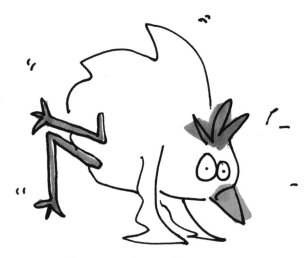

I exist only in the present.

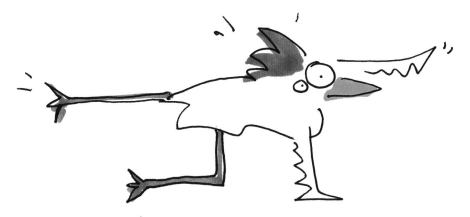

Lost Horizon Pose

The orientation of this pose speaks not only to the natural contradictions around us—the rising of the sun in the East, the setting of the sun in the West, for example—but also the spiritual contradictions of the wisdom of Eastern philosophies with the Western search for the new. This pose increases the stamina and focus necessary to find balance in these contradictions.

From an all-fours position, focus on a spot ahead of you and concentrate. Exhale and lift your right wing to point at that spot. Imagine a spot directly behind you—an opposite spot—and lift your right leg straight out to point directly at it, creating a horizontal body line. Extend your wingtips and toes as much as you can at either end to fully express the nature of life's contradictions, the conflicting pulls of existence. Inhale. Hold. Exhale back to all-fours. Repeat with the other side.

Legs Up the Fence

There is often a lesson to be learned from even the most troubling circumstance. This pose was the result of an unfortunate fall off a lofty fence post. But long after the stars have faded and the bruises healed, the restorative powers of this happenstance pose continue to rejuvenate tired feet and legs. It is, however, best started lying down, particularly for beginners.

Find a fence or wall you can rest against peacefully. Be wary of splinters: Many barn doors and fence posts have an elegant rustic appearance that can be problematic in a contact situation. Lie on the ground with your feet in the air, legs straight. Wiggle yourself close to the fence post or wall so your tail feathers touch it. Lie there with your eyes closed for several minutes. Stop if your legs fall asleep.

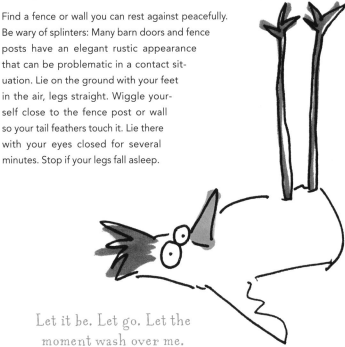

Let it be. Let go. Let the
moment wash over me.

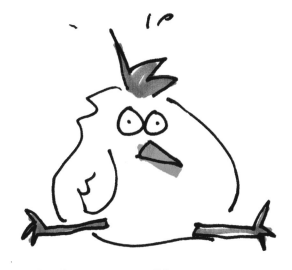

My heart is pure. My mind is open.
My body is glorious.

Thunder Thighs

This pose is a wonderful way to strengthen and stretch the inner-thigh area. Those with a strong degree of balance (or who don't have too much weight in the breast) might prefer to practice this pose standing up. In this case, try to touch the ground with the crest of your comb.

Sit on the ground and spread your legs as wide as they will go. Keeping your back straight and exhaling, lean forward and try to grasp your toes with your wingtips. Try to lay your breast feathers on the ground. Feel the ground's energy course through your breast. Inhale and hold. Exhale back up to sitting.

THE SHOVEL

Chicken was very clever, even as a chick. Her farmer had a precious shovel, a rare antique. Chicken happened to break this shovel and was greatly vexed. Hearing the footsteps of her farmer, she hid the broken shovel in the hay. When the farmer appeared, chicken asked: "Why do chickens have to die?"

"This is natural," explained the farmer. "Everything has to die and has just so long to live."

Chicken, producing the shattered shovel, added, "It was time for your shovel to die."

Flattened Chicken Poses

There are, perhaps, no more grounding experiences than these poses.

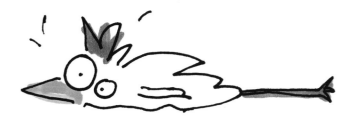

Why Did the Chicken Cross the Road?

For centuries this question has remained in our collective consciousness. We may not be able to answer why, but this pose is an ancient illustration of what.

Lie down on your breastbone and stretch your legs directly behind you, toes pointing in the opposite direction of your beak. Keep your beak pointed forward and pull your wings back parallel to your body. Keep the tension in your body and feel the hardness of the ground. Imagine yourself, but do not attempt this pose, on an actual road.

I drink deeply from the pail of joy.

Snake in the Grass

While life's challenges can get you down both spirtitually and physically, this pose is a reminder that, however prostrate, we all have the strength to rise up. No matter how enlightened we may seek to become, it is unlikely that the snake and the chicken will ever be friends. Yet still we may learn from its creeping ways and rise up out of the dirt.

Lie on your breastbone with your legs stretched out behind you, toes pointing. Place your wings on the ground under your shoulders— remembering to thank the creator for wings and shoulders. Tighten your tailfeathers and inhale. Push up with your wingtips and raise your beak and breastbone. Your legs remain on the ground. Exhale and release slowly down to the ground. Repeat.

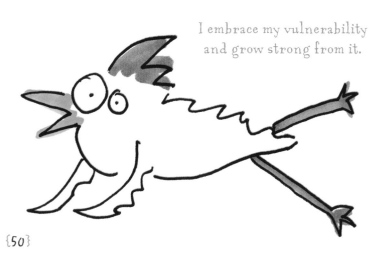

I embrace my vulnerability
and grow strong from it.

Twisted Chicken

The position and movement of this pose offers not only whole-body alignment, but also the opportunity for a nice little dust bath.

Lie on your back with wings outstretched. Stick your legs straight up in the air. Exhale and lower your legs to the right, keeping the rest of your body flat on the ground. Inhale and rotate your legs back up straight. Exhale and lower them to the left.

Waving Not Drowning

Though this is a position of vulnerability, great strength can be achieved from its simple extension.

Lie flat on your breastbone, with wings stretched down at your sides and legs pointing out behind you. Face your beak forward. Inhale and lift one leg behind you. Wave with your toes. Exhale and lower it to the ground. Repeat on the other side.

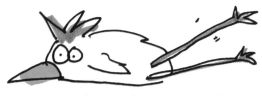

I am gloriously grounded.

Pigeon

It's probably bad karma to say so, but pigeons simply don't have the grace and dignity of chickens. They do, however, have extraordinary vertical elevation, thanks, perhaps, to this pose, which builds strength and flexibility in the buttocks and thighs.

Get down on all fours. Bring your left foot under your breast and extend your right leg straight out behind you. Put your head on the ground. Inhale and push your breast up with your wings until your wings are as straight as possible. Exhale out through your breast.

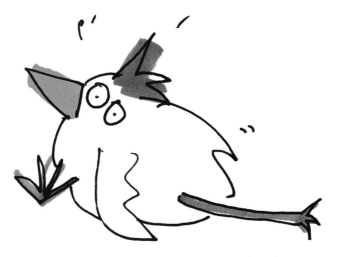

I allow my spirit to soar to great heights.

Count Your Chickens Before They Hatch Pose

In this unique pose, with feet high in the air and feathers firmly planted, one can be truly mindful of the effort and power and stress of egg laying. By raising your tail feathers high in salute to the sun, you give thanks for the eggs you have laid and all those yet to come, acknowledging your ability to reproduce.

Lie on your back on the ground with your wings down at your sides. Exhale and push your legs up high in the air. Feel the warmth and love from the atmosphere soak into your exposed underfeathers. Imagine your unlaid eggs thriving in this joy. Inhale and hold. Exhale and release back down, vertebra by vertebra.

Note: Only vertebrates can do this pose.

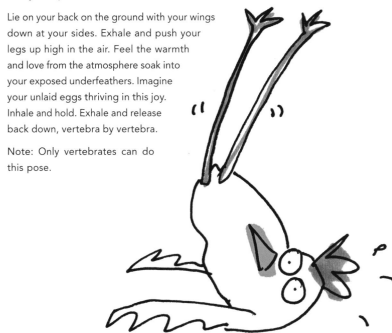

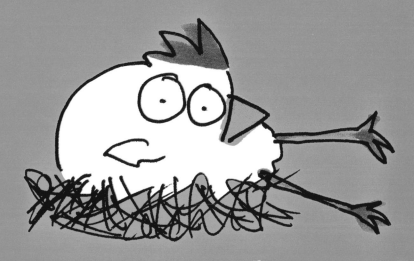

I exude bliss.

Sunnyside Up

Throughout our lives we tend to keep our soft underbelly down to the ground. While the earth is a powerful source of energy, the sun is also a source of great power. Lifting your belly to the sun is not only a great way to relieve tension in the back and neck; it also allows you to air out some of the underfeathers that seem to never get a chance to see the light of day.

Lie on your back with your legs bent. Gaze up into the sky as you inhale and thrust your backbone up, keeping your neck and wings on the ground. In this pose, you offer your childish energy to the heavens. Your weight is on your feet and shoulders. Hold. Exhale and lower, vertebra by vertebra.

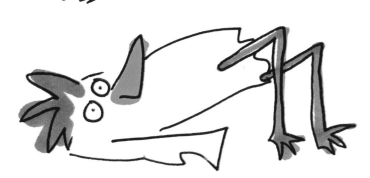

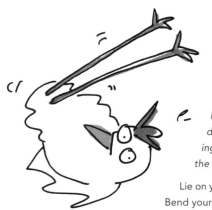

Over Easy

Chickens with high blood pressure, thyroid conditions, or glaucoma should avoid this position. For the rest of us, it promotes calmness and serenity, and does wonders for the skin. If you're feeling like a spring chicken, follow it up with the next two poses.

Lie on your back with your wings by your sides. Bend your knees up toward your breast and support your haunches with your wings. Straighten your legs and bend them back at a 45-degree angle over your head.

Over Hard

This is a natural extension for the adept at the Over Easy pose (see above). Those with less down on the neck may wish to support it and the shoulders with a soft cushion of hay.

Lie on your back with your wings by your sides. Bend your knees towards your breast, supporting your haunches with your wings. Keeping your head on the floor, extend your legs straight up, and lift from your egg-laying center. Gaze in wonderment at your toes above you.

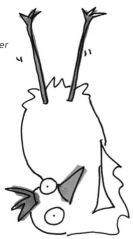

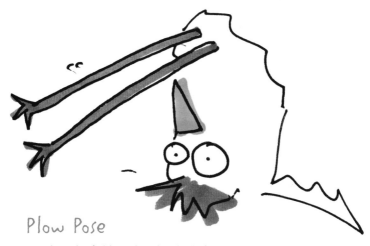

Plow Pose

"Look to the fields and in the sheds for inspiration," my mentor used to gently cluck. This pose comes from the human springtime ritual of plowing. It allows you to go beyond just scratching the surface and lets you tap into the life-giving richness of the soil of spring. And the tail-to-the-sky position allows a not-so-often-seen inner beauty to shine forth. This pose promotes serenity and earthiness.

Lie on your back, breast to the sun, wings down at your sides. Pressing down with your wings, exhale and lift your legs over and behind your head as far as they can go, keeping your legs straight and your beak straight up. You are the tool that awakens the earth! Inhale and hold. Exhale and slowly roll back to the ground, vertebra by vertabra.

I've Fallen and I Can't Get Up Pose

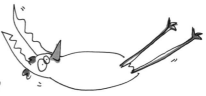

This is a pose I learned from the farmer's wife. She herself chose to practice it on a patch of ice, and accompanied it with loud arrhythmic chanting. While grounding is of the essence—in this pose as in life—unfrozen ground is preferable to prevent feathers sticking; and the position is, if anything, even more restorative and energizing when practiced in silence.

Lie flat on your back. As if you are pinned to the ground, inhale and reach up and out with your wings and feet in opposite directions. Your back remains leaden. Hold. Exhale and release.

Bad Bug

It happens to the best of us. You try to be choosy about the bugs you catch, but every once in a while a bad one sneaks in and wreaks havoc with your insides. What to do? Learn from it! This pose helps you release tension and, in aiding elimination, brings balance back to your whole body.

Lie on your back and sharply bring both knees into your breast feathers. Roll your eyes back into your head and exhale heavily. Hug your legs tightly with your wings and breathe deeply. Roll from side to side. Moving your head in the same direction as your body, expel any bad thoughts or memories.

Charlotte's Web

We farmyard creatures can only strive to emulate the spider. Her wisdom; her extraordinary patience and artistry as she spins her exquisite web; her matter-of-fact acceptance of the death of her prey—made all the more poignant by the fact that she will give her own life as she births her young. Hers is a very enlightened approach to existence. This pose, named in her honor, also does wonders for the thighs.

Lie on your back with legs straight. Exhale and lift your right leg and grasp it with your right wingtip. Pull your leg down to your shoulder, keeping it as straight as possible. From this pose you can admire the beauty of the spider's web up in the corner and the tone of your own drumstick. Inhale. Hold. Feel the energy flow into your legs. Exhale and release. Repeat with the other leg.

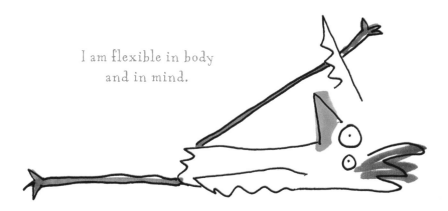

I am flexible in body
and in mind.

Chicken of the Sea Pose

You may have heard the expression "neither fish nor fowl." This pose embraces that contradiction, for can we not be both fish and fowl? Consider the much-maligned tuna. This pose opens the breastbone, strengthens the legs, and loosens the beak. All good for a chicken, either of land or of sea.

Lie on your back with your legs straight. Work your wings behind your back and clasp your wingtips together. Inhale as you heave your breastbone into the air and clench your legs. Hold for a few moments and exhale as you release back into a roosting position.

I rejoice in the beauty
and necessity of every
living thing.

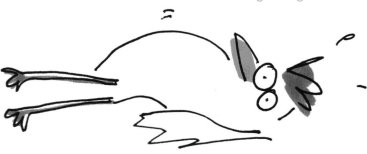

EMPTY MIND

A chick once asked Chicken: "If I haven't anything in my mind, what shall I do?"

Chicken replied: "Throw it out."

"But if I haven't anything, how can I throw it out?" continued the questioner.

"Well," said Chicken, "then carry it out."

CHICKEN ENTERS THE GATE

One day, as Chicken stood outside the gate, the farmer called to her, "Chicken, chicken, why do you not enter?"

Chicken replied, "I do not see myself as outside. Why enter?"

Roosting Chicken Poses

Chickens are great birds of a feather—we like to stick together. Whether it's in the barnyard, in the coop, or, if we're really lucky, up a tree, there's nothing we like better than a roost and a cluck together. All of these poses take on an extra dimension and special meaning when practiced in a roosting setting.

Poached Pose

At the end of a long day, when the dogs are barking, the farmer forgot the feed, the wind blew all the bugs away, and the eggs just aren't coming . . . When you are feeling toasted, roasted, and otherwise cooked . . . Relax in this Poached Pose and feel your energy heat up and recirculate.

Lie on your breastbone and stretch your legs behind you. Exhale deeply and reach your beak forward. Extend your right wing back at your side and your left wing at 12 o'clock. Feel the openness in your breast. Breathe deeply and feel yourself relax. Release your exterior shell. Imagine your muscles are warmed, soft, jiggly, and loose. Repeat with the other wing.

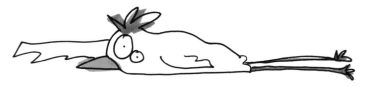

I offer my physical self to the forces of gravity.

Chick's Pose

Feeling like you could use a little protective shell around you to shield you from everyday stress and strain? Try Chick's Pose for a few minutes and soon you will be feeling fluffy all over.

From a kneeling position, widen your legs slightly and drop your tail feathers on your heels. Bring your breast and head toward the floor and release your wings behind you. Breathe into your lower back and relax into the innocence of chickness with each exhalation.

I am nurtured
and loved.

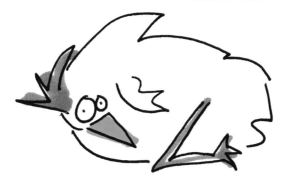

Chicken Little Pose

There is much about the sky that is scary. But we have nothing to fear except fear itself. Point to the sky with all your limbs and vehemently deny fear—it can help detox your system and shake the fear that crippled Chicken Little.

Lie on your back and raise your wings and legs into the air. Point at the sky and shake your wings, legs, and feet at it. Shake wildly for a count of 5. No fear! Exhale and relax your wings and legs back down to the ground.

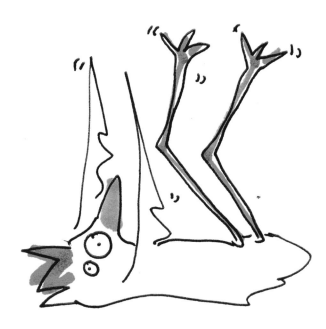

Boneless Chicken Pose

You know the feeling: You've taken a good grilling all day. Let your worries and your bones melt away in this relaxing pose.

Lie on your back with wings and legs flat on the ground, wings at a 90-degree angle to your body. Your body is sinking. Flesh and feather are at one with the earth. Breathe.

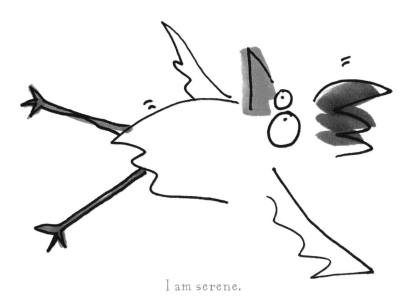

I am serene.

Egg Poses (Advanced)

These in-shell poses are very advanced, but there is much to be learned from their simple, embryonic elegance and innocence.

Just-Laid Pose

This pose requires total relaxation and quiet awareness. It is the first pose of creativity and mindfulness.

Lay on the most comfortable side of your shell. Hold. Reverse.

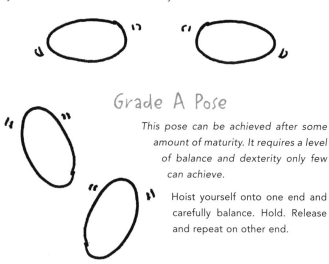

Grade A Pose

This pose can be achieved after some amount of maturity. It requires a level of balance and dexterity only few can achieve.

Hoist yourself onto one end and carefully balance. Hold. Release and repeat on other end.

I break out of the shell of myself and transcend.

Cracked Up Pose

This is the most mature of all egg poses. It teeters on the cusp of embryo and chicken. It is the essential life-affirming moment, one we spend the rest of our lives striving to recall.

When your legs are free for the first time, exhale and stretch them straight. Inhale and bend them under your shell. Exhale and straighten them to standing. Hold. If you feel balanced, extend one leg out. Come on out of your shell and greet the world! Repeat with the other leg.

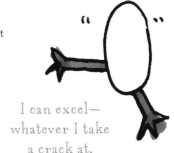

I can excel—
whatever I take
a crack at.

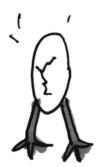

Morning has broken, like the first eggshell.

My feet are grounded.
My mind wanders.
My spirit soars.

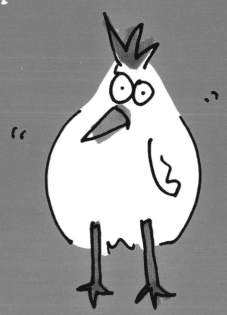

Bird in the Hand Poses

Traditionally, yoga is practiced alone. But for the chicken that is always open to new experiences, practicing with a partner offers yet more opportunities to delve within and become enlightened. There can be no self-consciousness, only self-awareness with these poses. Two chickens can create serenity between them and for each other through these intimate positions.

Double Chicken Squat

The common squat may seem a mundane pose to practice with a partner. But think about it. Together, two form a circle of wholeness through wing, leg, body, and ground, where energy can surge and heal.

Face your partner in Weathervane pose (see page 26). Reach forward and grasp wingtips. Inhale and hold. Exhale slowly as you both gently squat, pulling slightly on each other's wingtips. Feel the tension. When you both reach a full squat, hold. Feel the warmth of the energy that is multiplied by the partner's presence. Exhale back to standing. Thank your partner.

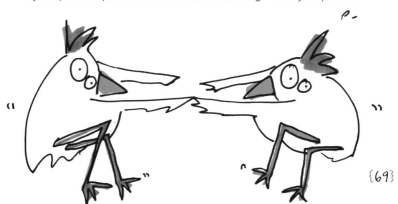

Up-Down Pose

When one chicken is up, the other is down. It's an ancient reality. This pose celebrates the seasons and rhythms of the chicken condition. The other great thing about this pose is that with your partner to guide you, it will help perfect your forward bends, which can be hard for chickens because of our ample breasts. This is a pose about letting go, but not letting go.

Sit on the floor with your legs straight out in front of you and your partner standing facing you, toes pointing outwards. Place your flexed feet against your partner's ankle bones. Grasp each other by the wingtips. Allow your partner to gently draw and stretch your arms forward.

Thank your partner and then trade positions. Be sure to check your partner's face for any sign of strain.

I allow my body
to articulate
eternal balance.

Double Dip

If this pose aids digestion and elimination when practiced alone, think what it can do for two!

Stand backbone to backbone with your partner in Weathervane pose (see page 26). Exhale and fold your bodies forward. Shimmy your body as close to your partner's as possible, preferably so that buttocks and tendons are touching. Grasp each other's ankle joints with your wingtips. Inhale and fully straighten your legs together. Exhale and pull your heads together as far as you can, as far as the combs touching if you're able. Hold for several breaths before slowly rising. Thank your partner.

Note: If you and your partner cannot bend over without bouncing your tailfeathers off each other, one of you should bend forward first, followed by the other, and then wiggle backwards until you assume the correct position.

I am in a constant state of fulfillment.

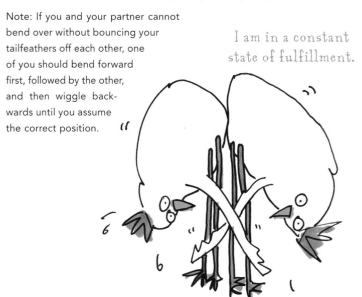

{71}

SLEEPING CHICKEN

One summer day the air had been so sultry that little chicken stretched her little chicken legs out, plopped her tailfeathers down, and went to sleep while the farmer was away.

Hours passed when, suddenly waking, she heard her farmer enter. But it was too late. There she lay, sprawled across the doorway.

"I beg your pardon, I beg your pardon," her farmer whispered, stepping carefully over chicken's body as if it were that of some distinguished guest. After this, chicken never slept again in the afternoon.

Fix-It Routines

Specific poses are terrific for unique stress points, but when you're really feeling plucked, you just need a little more. Thighs feeling tough? Neck frozen? Breast in need of a lift? Try these chicken fix-it routines and before you know it, you'll be feeling as fresh as a free-ranger. You'll find in these pages a combination of some earlier poses as well as a host of new ones.

Relief for Chicken Wings

When your wings are in a flap, this routine will extend your wingspan and take you to new heights.

Single Wingstand

Spiritually, this pose is akin to One Wing Flapping (see page 37). Physiologically, it is quite different: One wing bears the weight of your entire body, while the other floats above. This causes a rush of blood to your earthbound wing, while your skyward one strives for dizzying new heights. You won't believe how refreshing this is!

Start in an all-fours position. Straighten your legs out behind you in line with your back. Inhale. Rotate your body to the left, reach to the sky with your left wing, and stack your left foot on top of your right foot, like logs on the woodpile. Keep your body straight and balance. Hold for a few breaths and exhale down. Repeat on the other side.

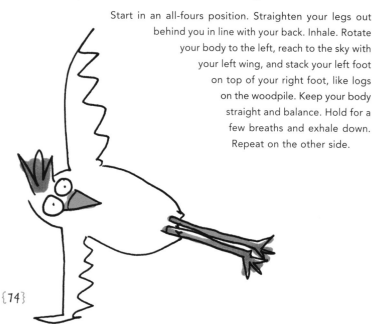

Floating Pretzel

A spurt of energy to refresh tired wings. Note: This is an advanced position. To make it extremely advanced, you may opt to flap your wings quickly and forcefully to lengthen the effect of floating.

Find a comfortable place to sit and place your tailfeathers directly on the ground. Fold your legs in front of you so that your left leg is resting on the ground and your right leg is resting on your left thigh, feet as close to your body as possible. Sit up straight and place your wingtips together over your head. Now exhale and push down with your wingtips until you lift your body off the ground. Inhale and immediately lift your wings overhead.

I am chicken, see me soar!

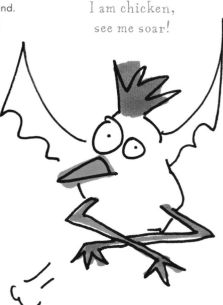

Air Traffic Control Pose

We've all known a goose or two that has met its unfortunate match with a departing 747. It is at such times that we chickens must humbly acknowledge the wisdom of the higher force that decreed us incapable of flight. This pose is inspired by such tragic events and is a way of giving back. When practiced with concentration, it can loosen wings and relieve tension, while also diverting wayward geese from danger.

Stand in Weathervane pose (see page 26). Inhale and sweep your right wing up and your left wing across your body. Hold. Look sympathetic, worried, and shocked. This facial expression helps dissipate the tension that can work its way into your beak area.

Exhale and sweep your wings in the reverse position. Repeat until you feel the tension fly off the ends of your wingtips.

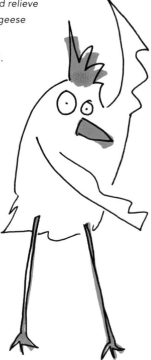

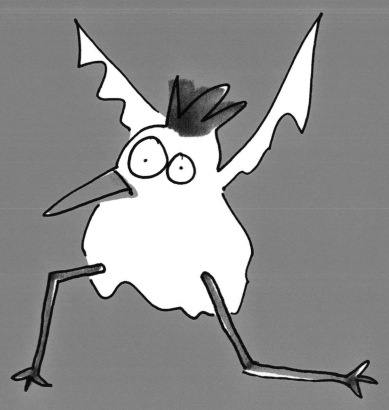

I am whole, calm,
  and perfect now.

Rx for Ruffled Feathers

Find yourself at the bottom of the pecking order? Not enough whole-grain cereal for breakfast? Been laying too many eggs lately? Let's face it: From time to time, we all get ruffled feathers. Try this routine the next time you feel as mad as a wet hen.

Funky Chicken

This moving meditation is a great way to free inhibitions and express your inner chick. Go shake a leg!

From a standing position, swing your wings up into the air to your right and give a tiny leap. Bring your knees high as you inhale. Feel the air lift your wings gently and lift away tension setting it free into the universe. Repeat on the other side.

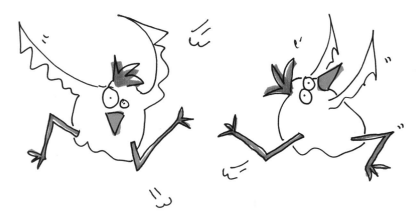

Proud Chicken Descending

What is more elegant than the chicken in flight? It is a masterpiece of nature and physics that our bodies can—even for a short time—keep ourselves in the air. It's a metaphorical meditation for keeping your thoughts lofty and your spirit light and free. Think of this pose as the manifestation of returning from the freedom of the air to the reality of the ground.

Start in Weathervane pose (see page 26) and exhale, raising your wings to the sky. Inhale and stretch farther—stand on your toes if possible, to feel the lift. Exhale and sweep your wings downward to the ground. Keep your legs straight while you reach for the ground. Inhale and hold. Exhale back to standing. Repeat on the other side.

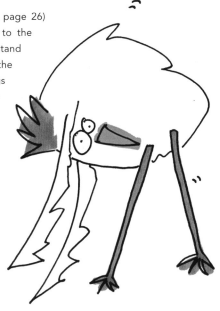

I enjoy each step on the path to enlightenment.

My Aching Chicken Feet

Poor chicken feet! A-pickin' and a-scratchin' all day! They silently carry all our weight and never complain about the abuse we expose them to. This quick routine is sure to put a spring in your step as it encourages your feet to worship the ground they walk on.

Leg Up Pose

This pose elongates tired, cramped legs and allows weary feet to refresh.

From Egg Laying Pose (see page 42), lift your right leg behind your head. Hold your leg with your wing. Breathe. Release and repeat with the other side.

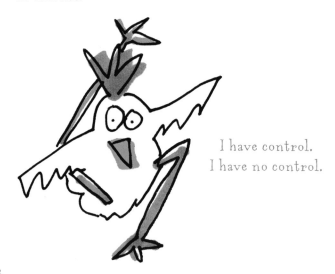

I have control.
I have no control.

Holding Toe Pose

Perhaps the most graceful of all poses, this toe grasper completes a sacred circle of wing to toe. In this position you can open a circuit of healing energy and recharge your tired feet.

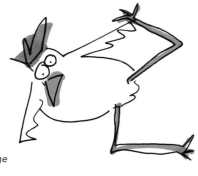

From an all-fours position, exhale and lift your left leg and reach back to grab it with your left wingtip. Pull taut. Hold for two breaths. Exhale back to all fours and repeat with the right side.

Cold Ground

It's a fact: There are places where feathers would be helpful. Inspired by the realities of winter, this pose allows you to lift and refresh one foot at a time.

I am balanced.

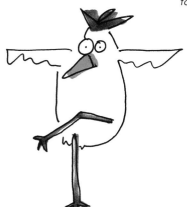

From Weathervane pose (see page 26), exhale and spread your wings out to the sides. Inhale and hold. Exhale and raise your left leg. Balance for a few breaths. Feel your toes spread and hold up the entire weight of your body, while the breeze refreshes the lifted foot. Exhale down to standing and repeat with the right leg.

Free Range Chicken

Feeling cooped up? No room to breathe? All caged-in inside? This routine will liberate you and have you feeling like a free ranger in no time.

Crouching Chicken Hidden Weasel

This pose originates in the age-old conflict between chickens and egg-stealing weasels. A traditional pose of active defense, this pose lengthens the spine and gets the energy flowing from beak to tail, bringing clear awareness and alertness to mind and body.

Begin in Chick's Pose (see page 63). Inhale and reach your wings forward on the ground in front of you. Exhale and lengthen one leg behind you and open your eyes as wide as possible. Breathe and hold. Exhale back to Chick's Pose. Repeat on the other side.

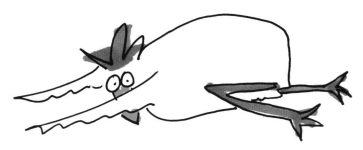

I have the power to transmute all my fears
into focused, calm happiness.

Take the Leap

To free yourself of the self-doubt and fear that can make you feel like a penned hen, you need, at times, to break out of your comfort zone.

From Weathervane pose (see page 26), inhale and leap off the ground as high as you can while keeping your wings and legs outstretched. Exhale when you land. A hopeful and open facial expression completes the pose.

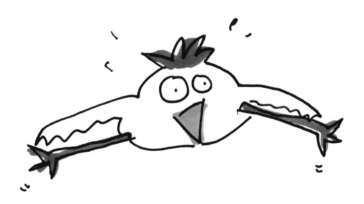

I listen to my body and I know
it is perfect in each moment.

Keep on the Sunnyside Up Routine

For the most part we live in a right-side-up world, but a change of scenery can do a body good. This upside-down routine can get the circulation flowing in places that never see the sun and give you a joyful new perspective on life.

Beak Up Backbend Pose

It's not often enough that we look straight up to the sky from a grounded position. This pose allows for a great stretch in the spine as well as a liberating view.

From a kneeling position, inhale and fling your wings back behind you in an attempt to grasp your toes. Look straight up. Breathe.

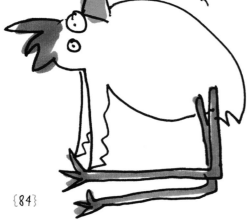

I am infinite.
My cup runs over.

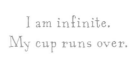

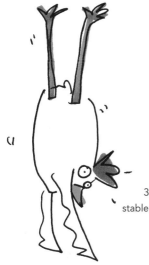

Wingstand

This one is an advanced pose that takes patience and grace. You may need the side of a barn to get up into the correct position.

From Grain on Ground Pose (see page 32), lift one leg into the air. When you feel stable, lift the other. Celebrate the awkwardness.

Ground Stretch

A super stretch for your entire body, this is very grounding and restorative, but also provides the opportunity for meditation on the skies above.

Lie down on your back and inhale. Exhale and stretch your wings back and over your head and your toes away from your body, so that the entire length of your physical being from tippy-toe to wingtip is in touch with the earth. Inhale back to resting.

I am fulfilled as a chicken.

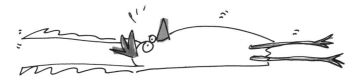

Routine for a Fried Chicken

We've all been there. Zapped of energy. On our last leg. Totally fried. Ready to drop on the nest for a rest. Instead, try these refreshing poses and you'll be on your feet and feeling like a spring chicken in no time.

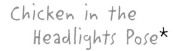

Chicken in the Headlights Pose*

The art of standing still is one that has been mastered by many creatures at crunch time. This meditation can be liberating and revitalizing.

Stand in Weathervane pose (see page 26). Exhale and take a step to the left. Hold for a count of 20. Concentrate on your surroundings. Focus on a single or double point of light. Breathe. On an inhale, return to center. Repeat on the other leg.

*CAUTION—do not attempt this pose on a road.

Thread the Needle

Sometimes inactivity can be as exhausting as overactivity. With too much to do and too little time, we find ourselves mired in schedules and stuck in a rut of our own making. This pose is symbolic of that condition—a reminder to move on and take giant steps through the tasks at hand in order to find a clearer path.

From the Worm! pose (see page 33), inhale and step your left leg under your left wing. Breathe. Exhale back to Worm! Repeat on the right side.

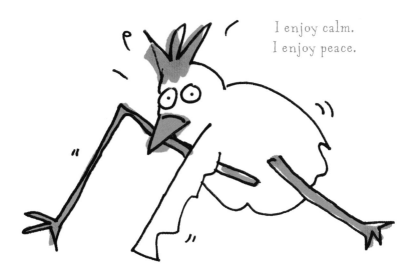

I enjoy calm.
I enjoy peace.

I'm Stuffed

Too much of a good thing can leave us all feeling a little dumpy and sluggish. With this fix-it routine, you will be feeling light as a feather in no time at all. Create a moment of tranquility in Wishbone pose (see page 27) to welcome this routine into being.

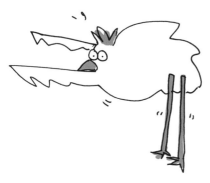

Forward Bend

A simple yet often frustratingly illusive pose, the Forward Bend encourages digestion.

From Weathervane pose (see page 26), inhale and reach the wings overhead and bend forward to make a right angle. Exhale back to standing.

Swimming Chicken

Though it is not often that a chicken will take to the water, this pose simulates the freedom associated with the water realm and is good for loosening a familiar tightness in the girth.

Standing in Forward Bend (see above), rotate the wings in a swimming motion while breathing. Exhale back to standing.

Sitting Duck

Borrowed from a feathered friend, this pose is a confidence builder as well as a get-up-and-go giver. By tapping into the vulnerability we all have inside, this kneeling/reaching pose brings together two essential opposite forces—earth and sky. By balancing between the two and feeling their pull, one can achieve a loosening stretch.

From a kneeling position, inhale and reach straight up overhead with your wings. Release your heavy thoughts. Exhale down to resting.

I am poultry in motion.

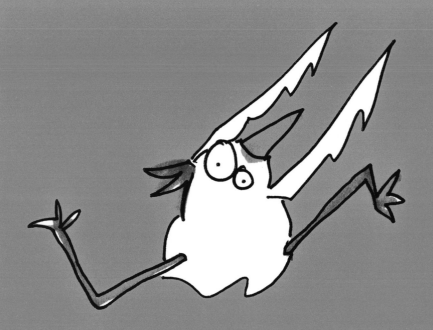

I am a deep well
into which I fling the
bucket of life.

Getting Off the Nest

There are days when all you want to do is roost. Whether we're feathering our nest, filling it with eggs, or just plain nesting, getting off it can be a problem. This routine gently pushes you off the nest and out into the real world with a feather-light touch.

You're Pulling Your Leg Pose

From Egg Laying Pose (see page 42), grasp each toe in a wingtip and pull. This pose should sting a bit. While the circulation is slightly cut off, you should be mindful of why sitting on your nest for great periods of time is not the wisest move.

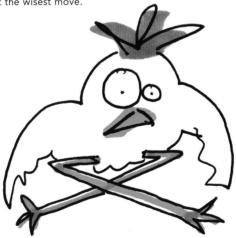

I receive the burn of enthusiasm.

Bent Leg Wing Lift

This balance and strength pose will get your heart pumping as you lift your body from the nest.

From Egg Laying Pose (see page 42), place your left leg under your body while straightening the right out over the nest rim. Slowly push down with your bent left leg until you are standing. Hold and breathe. Slowly descend back to the nest and repeat with the right leg.

Legs Over the Nest

Sometimes the boundaries of a nest can be debilitating. To extend physically first can help you go a long way in extending mentally and spiritually. In this pose you will awaken your legs.

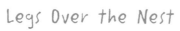

Sit comfortably with your legs in front of you. Inhale and exhale 3 times. On the last exhale, stretch your legs out as wide as you are able. Grab each big toe with a wingtip. Feel the pull. Hold. Inhale and imagine breaking through borders in your mind. Exhale back to sitting comfortably.

Bantam Strut

This pose says "Look at me! I am a chicken with gusto!" It energizes the whole body while it focuses energy outward and upward. With one long, outstretched leg still bound to the nest, the wings soar upward and touch the sky, reiterating your strong connection with creation, home, and family as well as the wild, untamed, unexplored wilderness of chickenhood.

From Weathervane pose (see page 26), exhale, bend your right knee, and lean over it with outstretched wings. Inhale and stretch even farther. Exhale back to Weathervane. Repeat on the other side.

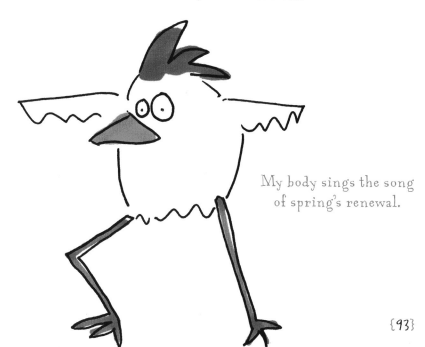

My body sings the song
of spring's renewal.

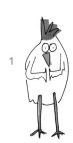
1

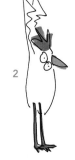
2

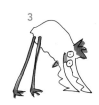
3

The Rooster's Sunrise Salutation

This is a perfect way to wake and greet the day. It was developed by roosters at the dawn of time and has been passed down from generation to generation. Roosters have made rather a show of this routine, but we can all enjoy the benefits of this practice.

{1} Start in Wishbone pose (see page 27) as the sun begins to make its appearance for the day. {2} Inhale and stretch your wings above your head. Stand on your toes as you lengthen your backbone to peek at the morning's first rays. You may opt to chant softly (see page 14) for the first time here. {3} Exhale and bend at the hips and reach your wings to

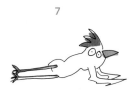
7

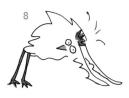
8

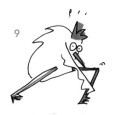
9

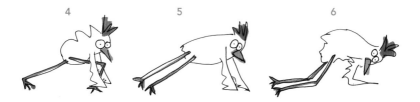

the ground in a sweeping motion. {4} Inhale and bend your right knee forward, stepping your left leg straight back into a lunge. {5} Exhale and bring your right leg straight back in alignment with your leg. Hold in this push-up position. Take a moment to view the bugs. {6} Inhale and lower your beak to the ground while keeping your tail feathers up. Slide your legs straight out behind you. Feel as one with the earth as you both welcome the sun's rays after the chill of night. {7} Exhale and slide your breastbone across the ground pushing your beak up and arching into Snake in the Grass pose (see page 50). Chant. {8} Inhale, tuck your toes under, and lift your tail feathers high into the growing sunlight as in Grain on Ground Pose (see page 32). {9} Exhale and step your left leg up back into a lunge. {10} Inhale and draw both legs up into a bend. {11} Sweep your wings up, out, and to the sun. {12} Finish the routine with a loud song of salutation and joy.

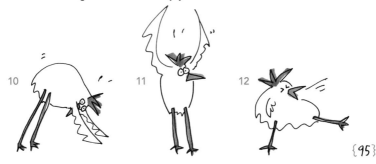

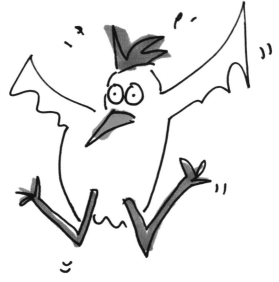

Spread Your Wings!

An Inspirational Message

This book encourages us to all look more deeply and to learn from those things that we might ordinarily overlook. There is hidden potential everywhere. To know yourself more deeply, perhaps even to know the true meaning of life—look to chickens. Join the flock. Cluck away the mundane pain and suffering of the daily grind and scratch beneath the surface. Take the time to stretch your wings, feel the wind in your feathers, and return to a simpler, more natural state. Discover your plucky inner chicken. Cackle with joy! Fly! Be free!